Juicing Recipes From The Rainbow

Juicing Your Way To Weight Loss, Health and Living a Lot Longer Drinking the Rainbow

Written by Soon Jang Wong

First Published, 2013

ISBN-13:978-0615918396 (WOS Publishing)

ISBN-10:0615918395

Printed in the United States of America

Table of Contents

Drink the Rainbow

The benefits of drinking your fruits and vegetables

"You better eat your vegetables!"

How many times has our parent's told us this when we were growing up—almost every meal, right? I know I heard this almost every meal time. I never liked eating my vegetables; they just paled in comparison to the macaroni and cheese or the chicken that was on my plate. Spinach and beets were the worst! The spinach looked like it came from the yard and the beets tasted like dirt. To this day, I still don't like beets.

"Put the cookies away; eat an apple if you're hungry."

That line was always followed by some whining and pouting on the kid's part. The true test would be the kid actually ate the apple. For me,

I never ate the apple so I would go without a snack. The only way I would eat an apple was if I had French dressing to go with it. Yes, I'm aware that is a weird and maybe disgusting combination. Don't judge, I was a kid!

Luckily, now that I am an adult my taste buds have changed and I like my fruits and vegetables. As much as I may like them I've got to admit that I don't eat them as much as I should. Like most people, I don't come anywhere close to the daily recommendations. As adults, we are supposed get anywhere between of 3 to 5 servings of both fruits and vegetables. That's a lot of produce!

An excellent way to get the nutrients that are found in fruits and vegetables is to juice—you should still eat some fruits and vegetables throughout the day though. Now mind you, there are no stark differences between the benefits of juicing and eating the fruit and vegetable. You are still getting the nutrients that are necessary for your body to function well.

Truth be told, eating a whole piece of fruit or vegetable is the best option, however drinking your daily fruit and vegetable requirements is easily the next best thing. Perhaps the only thing you aren't getting when you juice is the fiber from the whole produce. When juicing, the fiber is found in the pulp (the left over products from when you juice). Don't throw the pulp away though. You can incorporate the pulp into foods. The fruitier pulps can be used in baking and the more vegetable based pulps can be added to sauces and soups.

So you may be asking why I should start juicing my fruits and vegetables. Well, as I mentioned before, you'll be able to get all the benefits from getting the daily recommendation in one glass. Since the nutrients are found in the juice that's been extracted from those fruits and vegetables, your body is able to absorb those nutrients better. It also allows your body to take a break from its usual routine of breaking down fiber. Think of juicing as giving your body a lighter work load.

As you read the following pages, you'll see a reoccurring theme when it comes to the benefits that the various fruits and vegetables can do for you. Juicing your fruits and vegetables is said to help improve your immune system, reduce the risk for heart disease and lower your cholesterol. It also can help improve your vision, strengthen your bones and teeth; they can also help your hair and skin to look healthier. Some say that the nutrients found in plant based foods help prevent certain types of cancer! While there aren't many proven scientific studies that prove these popular beliefs, it is no secret that plant based foods are some of the best things that you could put into your body. These are just some of the benefits.

As you read more, you will find what colors offer what benefits to the body. However, you'll see that not one color group is more important or beneficial than another, but you will that they all have common properties. When eaten together, you'll begin to feel better. The brighter juices—like the yellow, red, and orange—often may lift your mood too.

There are some things that you should keep in mind when you juice though. You should always wash your produce thoroughly. You don't want dirty mixing in with your juice! It may seem like a common sense thing, but sometimes we forget, I know I do. Juicing is not meant to be a meal replacement. It should go along with a healthy diet. It is ideal to drink the juice on an empty stomach and eat 30 minutes after you drink. You can also have your juice about two hours after you eat. Try to only make the juice you plan on drinking right away. When you drink juice that was freshly made has the highest concentration of nutrients. The moment that the juice hits the air, it starts to oxidize and loses its potency. You can store juice if it is filled to the very top in an air tight container. There can be no air gap. You also want to keep your juice cold because the bacteria can grow rapidly if the juice is at room temperature. Along with keeping your juice cold, you want to wash your juicer or blender very well and for the same reason—to keep the bacteria away. We don't want to get sick; we're trying to get healthy after all!

Blue and Purple

Improve mineral absorption, powerful antioxidants

Two of the darkest colors in the color wheel, you wouldn't think they had much to offer in the health benefit department. Oh, but they do! Truth be told, these dark beauties are packed full of benefits! If you hadn't noticed by now, fresh fruits and vegetables are full of antioxidants. These are no different. Blueberries are often said to be a super fruit due to high levels of antioxidants in them. Along with the antioxidants this color family has in them, they also help prevent heart disease and type 2 diabetes.

Blue and purple foods have other benefits to them too. They contain anthocyanins (sound familiar?) that can help prevent urinary tract infections. Anthocyanins are also found in red foods and like the red foods we've talked about, the blues and purples can help the circulatory system and prevent certain types of cancer. It is also thought that they can improve your balance, vision, skin, and coordination as you age; however, more research has to be conducted to prove these claims.

Some common ingredients in blue/purple juices are:

- Plums
- Blueberries
- Blackberries
- Red Cabbage
- Beets
- Grapes

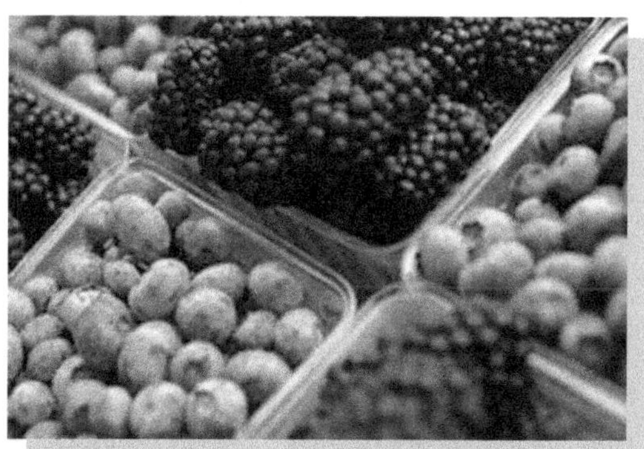

Blackberry and Grape Juice

Ingredients:

2 cups blackberries

2 cups black or purple grapes

2" piece of ginger root

Directions:

Wash Berries
Juice

Apple, Beet and Carrot Juice

Ingredients:

1/2 medium beet

2 fresh carrots

1 apple

Directions:

Core apple
Juice

Blueberry, Apple, and Romaine Juice

Ingredients:

3 cups blueberries

1 cup raspberries

2 Romaine hearts

3 Fuji apples

Directions:

Clean berries and romaine

Core apple

Juice

Red Cabbage, Apple, and Carrot Juice

Ingredients:

2 Celery Stalks

1/2 Carrot

1 Cucumber

1 Handful of Spinach

1/2 Lemon Peeled

1 Beet Sliced

1 Granny Smith Apple

1/4 Head of Red Cabbage

1" of Fresh Ginger Root

Directions:

Peel Cucumber and Lemon
Core Apple
Slice Beet
Juice

Orange

Prevent cancer and promote collagen growth

Let's go back to art class in school for a second. When learning our colors, we learned that red and yellow makes orange Simple stuff right? So it shouldn't surprise you that orange foods have the same qualities as red and yellow foods. Just like the other two colors, orange foods have beta-carotene in them. We also know that the beta-carotene is converted to Vitamin A and the benefits that the vitamin does for our bodies.

You know when you're sick, people tell you to drink plenty of orange juice? Well we know that orange juice and other citric fruits are full of vitamin C. This vitamin has a lot of benefits! It helps prevent and treat cold symptoms, helps lower cholesterol, prevent heart disease, prevent some cancers and it also used to treat depression. To list all the benefits would be a whole section for itself.

Interesting fact: Have you ever heard of the term "scurvy" in pirate stories? It's a real condition that affects anyone with a vitamin C deficiency. Scurvy was most common in people who sailed over-seas in the past. Fresh fruits and vegetables only last so long, and so when those products were gone, so were the sources for vitamin C.

Some of the fruits and vegetables that are rich in these nutrients include:

- Carrots
- Yams
- Butternut Squash
- Cantaloupe
- Pumpkin
- Sweet potato
- Peaches
- Apricots

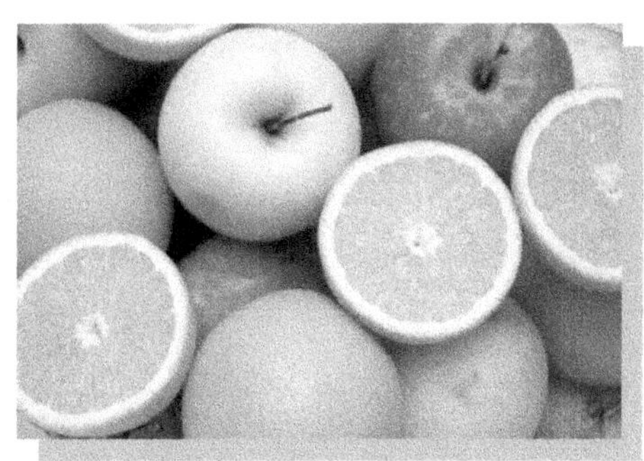

- Nectarines
- Tangerines

Carrot, Pineapple, and Orange Juice

Ingredients:

2 medium carrots

1/2 pineapple

2 oranges

Directions:

Remove orange from rind

Clean pineapple

Juice

Cantaloupe, Orange, and Ginger Juice

Ingredients:

1 cantaloupe

1 tbsp. raw ginger

1 orange

Directions:

Remove rind from orange and cantaloupe

Remove seeds from cantaloupe

Juice

Grapefruit, Apple, and Carrot Juice

Ingredients:

1 small grapefruit

1 apple

2 medium carrots

1/2 small lemon

1/4 inch of ginger room

Directions:

Peel grapefruit and lemon, remove seeds

Core apple

Juice

Spicy Orange, Apple, and Ginger Juice

Ingredients:

1 large orange

½ lemon

1 apple

1 tbsp. ginger root

(Optional) dash of cayenne pepper

Directions:

Peel orange and lemon

Core apple

Juice apple

Add cayenne pepper after juicing

Carrot, Apple, Celery and Grapefruit Juice

Ingredients:

4 large carrots

4 celery stalks

1 golden delicious apple

1 gala apple

1 grapefruit

Directions:

Core apples

Peel grapefruit

Juice

Mango, Pineapple, and Orange Juice

Ingredients:

1 mango

2 small carrots

1/2 pineapple

1 orange

Directions:

Peel mango and orange

Remove pit from mango

Remove rind from pineapple

Juice

Orange, carrot, Apple, Ginger Juice

Ingredients:

1 apple

4 carrots

1 small cucumber

1/2 in ginger root

Directions:

Core apple

Peel cucumber

Juice

Peach, Mango, Orange Juice

Ingredients:

1 mango

2 peaches

1 orange

1 plum

Directions:

Peel mango and orange

Remove pits from peaches, mango, & plum

Juice

Peppers and Apple Juice

Ingredients:

2 yellow peppers

2 orange peppers

1 red pepper

2 Fuji apples

Directions:

Core apples

De-seed peppers

Juice

Apple, Carrot, Grape and Beet Juice

Ingredients:

2 carrots

2 apples

2 dozen grapes

1 yellow beet

A small handful of baby spinach

Directions:

Core apples

Clean spinach

Juice

Yellow

Helps your heart, vision quality, digestion, and immune system

There's an old adage that we eat with our eyes. Food always looks more appetizing when they are presented nicely. There isn't much of a way to make a liquid more appealing and appetizing, however the color can improve your mood.

When the color yellow is used for interior decorating, it is seen as cheery and happy. When someone wears yellow clothing, they seem happier and maybe even more cheerful. By going with that theory, drinking yellow can also offer the same effect. Now, I'm not saying that drinking yellow is like drinking sunshine and will instantly lift your spirits and you'll be happier, but it's still a nice thought.

Some of the benefits from eating yellow include a large boost of vitamin C and antioxidants (sound familiar?). The yellow foods have been suggested to help improve your heart health, vision clarity, digestion and your immune system. Along with these, your skin will be healthier, wounds will heal quicker and bones and teeth will be stronger.

Some of the fruits and vegetables that's full of these nutrients include:

- Pineapple
- Lemons
- Squash
- Starfruit
- Corn
- Yellow Beets
- Yellow Peppers
- Mango

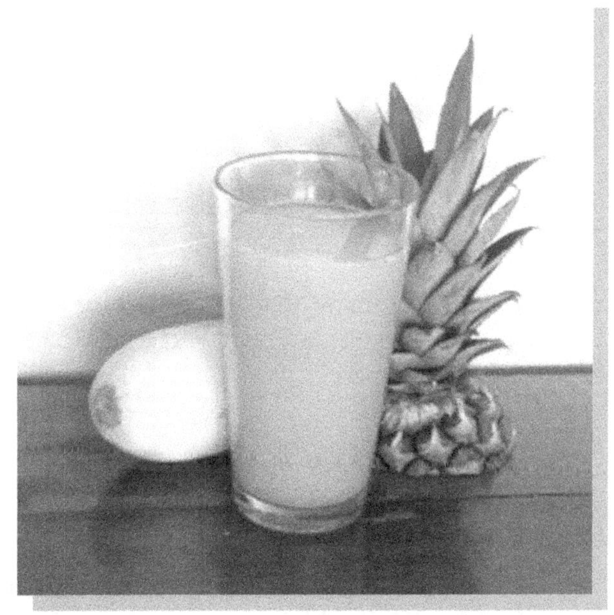

Mango, Orange and Yellow Pepper Juice

Ingredients:

2 mangoes

1 orange

1 yellow pepper

Directions:

Peel mango and orange

De-see pepper

Juice

Peach, Pear, and Carrot Juice

Ingredients:

2 peaches

1 large pear

2 yellow carrots

1 cup of green seedless grapes

A pinch of cinnamon

Directions:

Pit the peaches

De-seed pepper

Juice

Sprinkle with cinnamon if desired

Pineapple and Yellow Pepper Juice

Ingredients:

1 yellow pepper

1 yellow squash

1 pineapple

Directions:

De-seed the pepper

Remove rind from pineapple

Juice

Apple, Cucumber, and Squash Juice

Ingredients:

1 apple

2 cucumbers

1 yellow squash

1 yellow pepper

3 stalks of fennel

1 lemon

Directions:

Peel vegetables

De-seed pepper

Juice

Grapefruit, Pineapple, Apple Juice

Ingredients:

2 grapefruits

1 pineapple

2 yellow delicious apples

1/4 watermelon

Directions:

Peel grapefruit

Core apple

Juice

Apple, Carrot, and Yellow Beet Juice

Ingredients:

1 apple

4 carrots

2 yellow beets

1/4 inch ginger root

Directions:

Core apple

Juice

Lemon, Lime and Apple Juice

Ingredients:

1 lemon

1 lime

2 pears

2 green apples

2 carrots

2 cups chopped cabbage

Directions:

Peel lemon and lime

Core apple

Juice

Cucumber, Lemon, and Yellow Pepper Juice

Ingredients:

1 cucumber

1 yellow pepper

1/4 lemon

Directions:

Peel cucumber

De-seed pepper

Juice

Mango, Yellow Pepper and Cucumber Juice

Ingredients:

1 mango

1/2 cucumber

1/4 yellow pepper

1/4 jalapeno

2 green onions

1/4 cup cilantro

1/2 lime

Directions:

Remove seeds from jalapeno for less heat

De-seed yellow pepper

Peel mango and cucumber

Remove pit from mango

Juice

Orange, Pineapple, and Banana Smoothie

Ingredients:

2 oranges

1 pineapple

1 banana

2 – 4 ice cubes

Directions:

Peel banana, orange, and pineapple

Juice orange and pineapple

Combine juice with banana and ice in blender

Blend until smooth

Green

Energize, Detox and Improve Your Immune System

We are always being told that we need antioxidants in our diets; however, no one tells us exactly what antioxidants do. Well, in short they boost our immune system and can clean the blood from toxins. Also researchers believe that antioxidants have anti-aging properties and can prevent age related illnesses and diseases. Sounds pretty good right? Who doesn't want to maintain their youthful health and glow for as long as possible? I know I certainly do!

One way you can do this is by making and drinking green juice. You may have seen people touting the benefits of green juice and saying how it's changed their lives. Changing your life? That may be a bit of a stretch, but the green juice does offer health benefits that you don't always get.

When you eat the vegetable, your body lacks the proper enzymes that your body needs to break the cell walls of the vegetable. By juicing or blending your green vegetables, you are able to get all the nutrients from the leafy greens. This allows your body to absorb the nutrients much more efficiently.

Leafy greens contain chlorophyll. This stuff is pretty close to the molecular make up of our red blood cells. The only difference is it has magnesium at the core and our blood is rich with iron. What that means is it gives us energy and it also helps to clean the blood. Think of it as giving your kidneys a little rest. Not only does green juice contain chlorophyll to clean your blood, it also has fiber and other nutrients that will clean out your digestive system. Who needs laxatives when you can drink a good tasting juice or smoothie instead?

There are various nutrients that are found in green vegetables, and they are called phytonutrients. These nutrients boost your immune system and help to keep your cells intact and keep you healthy.

So, now that you know the benefits of green juices, let's make some!

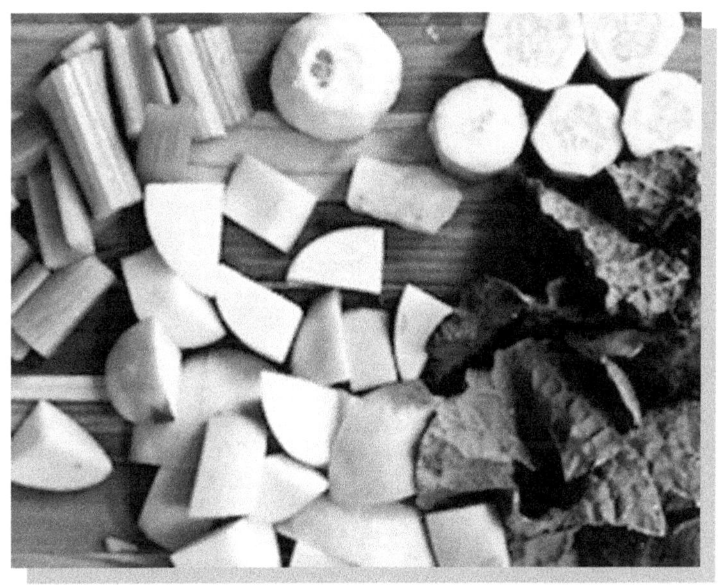

"Mean, Green Juice"

(As seen on Fat, Sick, and Nearly Dead)

Ingredients:

1 cucumber

4 celery stalks

2 green apples

6-8 kale leaves

½ lemon

1 tbsp. ginger

Directions:

Peel lemon and cucumber

Juice

Green Apple Juice

Ingredients:

2 green apples

1/2 cucumber

1 handful of romaine

2 handfuls of wheat grass

2 celery stalks

3 handfuls of kale

2 handfuls of spinach

1 lemon

Directions:

Core apples

Peel cucumber and lemon

Juice

Kiwi and Pear Juice

Ingredients:

1 pear

5 – 6 kiwi

1 large cucumber

2 celery stalks

6 leaves of romaine

1 handful of spinach

Directions:

Core pear

Peel kiwi and cucumber

Juice

Cucumber, Pear, and Honeydew Juice

Ingredients:

1 cucumber

2 celery stalks

2 pears

1/3 honeydew

8 kale leaves

1 lemon

1 inch ginger root

Directions:

Peel honeydew, lemon and cucumber

Core pears

Remove seeds from honeydew

Juice

Kale, Pineapple and Mint Juice

Ingredients:

1 cucumber

1 green apple

1 small pineapple

3 kale leaves

Small bunch of mint

1/2 lemon

Directions:

Peel cucumber, pineapple, and lemon

Core apple

Juice

Apple and Watermelon Juice

Ingredients:

2 green apples

5 swiss chard leaves

2 celery stalks

1 bunch of parsley

1 lemon

1/4 inch ginger root

Watermelon rind

Directions:

Peel lemon

Core apple

Use only the watermelon rind

Juice

Beet Greens and Cabbage Juice

Ingredients:

7 Beet greens

1/2 medium head of green cabbage

1 stalk of fennel (including leaves)

1 cucumber

Directions:

Use only beet greens, no beet

Peel cucumber

Juice

Fennel, Green Cabbage, and Sweet Potato Juice

Ingredients:

1/2 head of fennel

1/4 head of green cabbage

1 green bell pepper

3 stalks of celery

1 cucumber

1 sweet potato

1 inch ginger root

Directions:

Use entire fennel

De-seed pepper

Peel cucumber

Juice

"Dr. Oz Green Juice"

(As seen on Dr. Oz Show)

Ingredients:

2 cups spinach

1/2 cucumber

1/4 head of celery

1/2 bunch parsley

1 bunch mint

3 carrots

2 apples

1/4 orange

1/4 lime

1/4 lemon

1/4 pineapple

Directions:

Peel cucumber, lemon, lime, and orange

Core apple

Juice

“Shamrock” Juice

Ingredients:

1/2 frozen banana

1 cup spinach

1 cup coconut milk

2 drops pure vanilla extract

2 – 3 drops peppermint extract

Directions:

Blend ingredients together in a blender

Red

Improve the health of your joints, heart, and blood.

Lycopene and anthocyanin are pigments that gives fruits and vegetables their vibrant red color; and by drinking red juices, you are helping your circulatory system and keep a steady blood pressure. These pigments also have been known to lower cholesterol levels. Not only do they help your blood pressure and heart health, but researchers have shown that by eating produce with anthocyanin pigments in them, you are promoting healthy cell growth and division. The healthier your cells are means that you lessen the chances you could develop cancer. Fellas, you may want to bulk up on the reds because the main cancer they can prevent is prostate cancer.

Beta-carotene is another component that these ruby beauties have in them that our bodies use. The beta-carotenes are converted into vitamin A; and this vitamin helps support our immune system by strengthening our white blood cells. Along with the anthocyanin pigments, vitamin A also promotes healthy cells and helps to prevent cancer. The immune system also gets a boost from the vitamin C that is found in the produce also.

Some common ingredients in red juices are:

- Red cabbage
- Beet roots
- Tomatoes
- Strawberries
- Red Peppers
- Apples

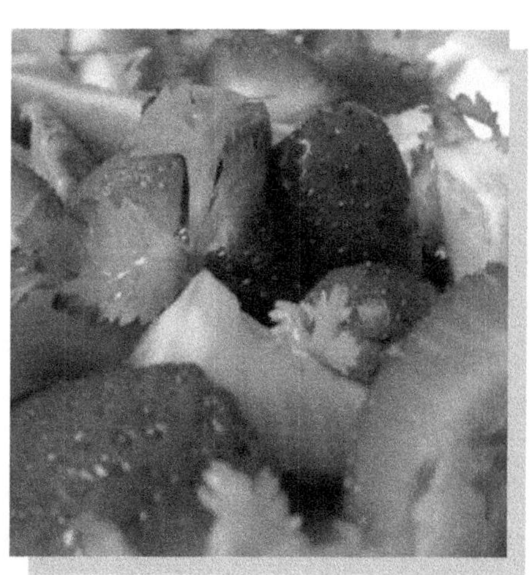

Beets, Red Pepper, and Watermelon Juice

Ingredients:

1 cup red beets

1 red pepper

2 cups watermelon

1 cup strawberries

1 cucumber

1 lime

Directions:

De-seed pepper

Remove stems from strawberries

Peel cucumber and lime

Juice

Beet, Carrot, and Strawberry Juice

Ingredients:

1 beet

2 carrots

6 strawberries

1 cup grapes

1 apple

Directions:

Remove stems from strawberries

Core apple

Juice

Celery, Apple, Carrot and Beet Juice

Ingredients:

1 small beet

2 large carrots

1 stalk of celery

1 apple

Directions:

Core apple

Juice

Strawberry, Mango, and Cucumber Juice

Ingredients:

1 apple

2 red cabbage leaves

2 medium carrots

1 cucumber

1 mango

1 bunch of parsley

1 cup of strawberries

Directions:

Core apple

Peel cucumber and mango

Remove pit from mango

Remove stems from strawberries

Juice

Spicy Tomato Cucumber Juice

Ingredients:

4 ripe tomatoes

4 cucumbers

1 small jalapeno pepper

2 celery stalks

2 basil leaves

Directions:

Peel cucumbers

De-seed jalapeno

Juice

Red Grape, Kale, and Red Cabbage Juice

Ingredients:

1 cup red grapes

1 cup kale

1 cup red cabbage

1 banana

1/2 cup ice

Directions:

Remove banana peel

Blend all ingredients in a blender

Blueberry, Blood Orange, and Beet Juice

Ingredients:

1 cup blueberries

3 blood oranges

1 grapefruit

1 small beet

Directions:

Peel oranges and grapefruit

Juice

Tomato and Basil Juice

Ingredients:

8 large tomatoes

1 large handful of basil

3 green onions

1 small garlic clove

Black pepper to taste

Directions:

Juice all ingredients together

Add pepper at the end for flavor

Beet, Strawberry, Pomegranate Juice

Ingredients:

1 beet

1 banana

2 stalks of celery

4 kale leaves

Small bunch of mint

1 cup water

1/2 cup pomegranate juice

1/4 cup blueberries

7 strawberries

1 lemon

1 lime

Directions:

Peel banana, lemon and lime

Blend all ingredients in a blender until smooth

Red Velvet Beet Smoothie

Ingredients:

1 cup vanilla Soy milk

1/2 cup Greek yogurt

2 medium beets

1 tbsp. Dutch cocoa powder

2 packets of sweetener

Direction:

Roast beets until tender, let cool.

Blend all ingredients

Difference in Juicers

Centrifugal Juice Extractor or Cold Press Juicer

If you're new to juicing, you may think that all juicers were created equal. Unfortunately, they are not. There are two types of juicers that you need to know about, Centrifugal Juice Extractors (known from now on as CJE) and cold press juicer (or also known as a masticating juicer).

CJE juicers are found in most homes. Using centrifugal force, a metal blade inside the device spins at high speeds and pushes the juice from the flesh. The juice and the pulp are separated and put into two different containers. Be forewarned though, the CJE heats up during the juicing process. Cold press juicers work by crushing the fruit or vegetable and then press it to get the most juice yield. The cold press is so aptly named because the device doesn't heat up nearly as much as the CJE.

If you are looking to begin juicing for health benefits, you should purchase a slow press juicer. While they are more expensive, the will give you the maximum amount of nutrients possible from the fruit and vegetables. The CJE is more recommended for those who plan to use the juices for cooking and aren't too concerned with nutrient intake.

Juicers at a Glance

	Centrifugal Juicer	Cold Press Juicer
Nutrient Retention	Due to the heat, this juicer breaks down nutrients, so they aren't as potent.	There is very little heat, so the potency of the nutrients are almost like you are eating the fruit/vegetable fresh
Press Green Leafy Vegetables?	It is possible, however not very efficient.	This juicer works very well for juicing leafy greens.
Process Nuts?	No	Yes, it works well for nuts. Instead of buying almond milk, you can essentially make your own.
Noise Level	Very noisy. Comparable to a blender.	Quiet.
Speed	Same Speed	Same Speed

Pulp	Some pulp	A lot of pulp
Price	Less Expensive	More Expensive

Centrifugal Juice Extractor

(Information Provided by Amazon.com)

Breville BJE200XL Compact Juice Fountain 700-Watt Juice Extractor

List Price - $130

Rating – 4.5 Stars

Description:

The juicer comes with a heavy-duty compact juice fountain with a center blade assembly. The 700 watt motor operates at 14,000 rpm (rotations per minute). The feeding tube is 3 inches in diameter and is positioned in the center of the device. There is a stainless steel micro-mesh filter to prevent pulp and seeds from getting into the juice.

The juicer has dishwasher safe parts and there is also a custom cleaning brush included.

There is a one year limited warranty on this product.

(Information Provided by Amazon.com)

Breville JE98XL Juice Fountain Plus 850-Watt Juice Extractor

List Price - $199

Rating – 4.5 Stars

Description:

This juicer has a 3 inch feeding tube and runs off of an 850 watt dual speed motor. The cutting disk is made of stainless steel and it creates fast results while juicing. There is a safety locking arm and there's an overload protection LED. The pulp collector can hold a substantial amount of refuse.

There are dishwasher safe parts and it comes with a 1 liter juice pitcher, filter basket, and a cleaning brush.

This juicer has a 1 year limited warranty.

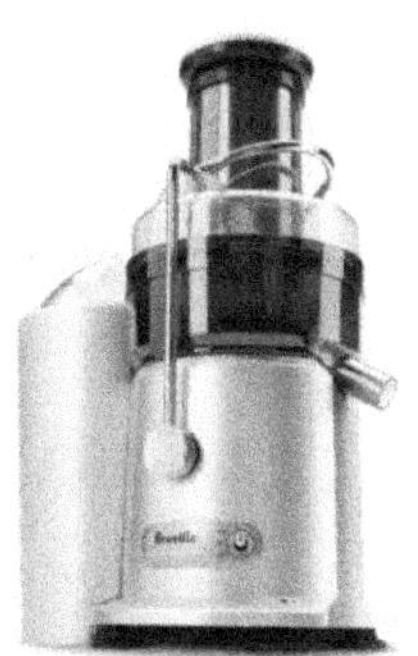

(Information Provided by Amazon.com)

Black & Decker JE2200 400-Watt Fruit and Vegetable Juice Extractor with Custom Juice Cup

List Price - $39.99

Rating – 4 Stars

Description:

This juicer has a 400 watt motor with a stainless steel cutter. This juicer will be able to juice and strain your fruits and vegetables easily. There is a large pulp container build into the juicer for saving space on the counter top.

This comes with a custom juicing cup and there are dishwasher safe parts.

This juicer comes with a 2 year, limited warranty.

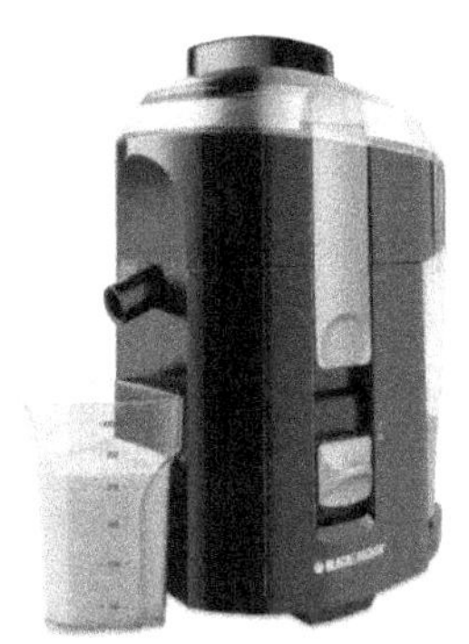

(Information Provided by Amazon.com)

Hamilton Beach 67608 Big Mouth Juice Extractor, Stainless Steel

List Price - $69.99

Rating – 4 Stars

Description:

This juicer boasts to make up to 24% more juice than other leading juicers. You can juice whole fruits quickly without having to do much prep work. The juicer has an 800 watt motor that is able to extract juice from all sorts of produce. The large pulp container allows you to save the pulp for any recipe.

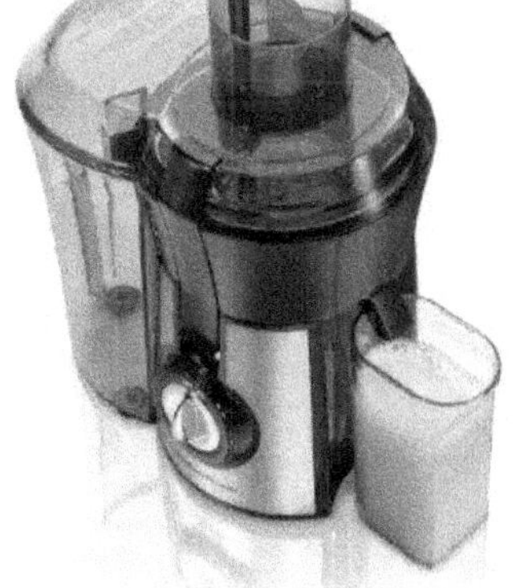

The juicer has dishwasher safe parts.

(Information Provided by Amazon.com)

Breville 800JEXL Juice Fountain Elite 1000-Watt Juice Extractor

List Price - $399

Rating – 4.5 Stars

Description:

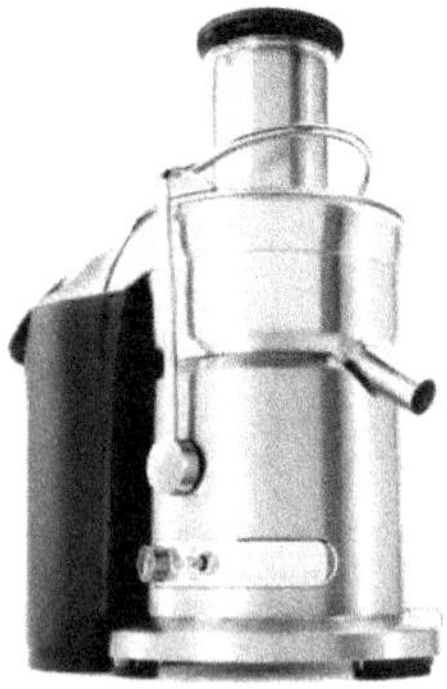

This juicer has a 1,000 watt motor with 2 different speeds--the high runs at 13,000 rpm and the low runs at 6,500 rpm. The cutting disk is made out of titanium and the juicer itself is made from die-cast steel. There is a 3 inch wide feeding tube.

The juicer comes with a pulp container, a pitcher to store the juice, and a recipe book/manual. There are dishwasher safe parts.

Cold Press (Masticating) Juicers

(Information Provided by Amazon.com)

Omega j8006 Center Juicer (Commercial Grade)

List Price – $390

Rating – 4.5 Stars

Description:

This juicer is easy to use and it runs at a low speed of

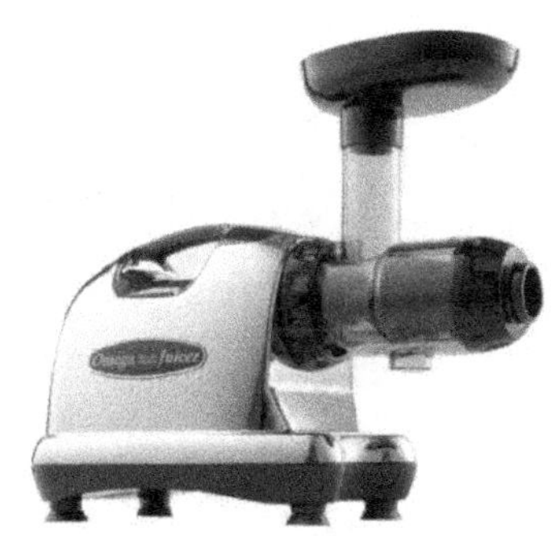

80 rpm which reduces foaming, clogging or built up heat. There is a high juice yield and an auto pulp-ejection function to allow for continuous juicing. There is a dual juicing system which allows for quiet operation.

This juicer comes with a 15 year warranty.

(Information Provided by Amazon.com)

Omega J8003 Nutrition Center Single-Gear (Commercial Grade)

List Price – $300

Rating – 4.5 Stars

Description:

This is a commercial grade juicer with a 1/3 HP single phase induction motor. There is a dual stage juicing system and runs at a low speed of 80 rpm. This reduces foaming, clogging, and heat from building up.

This juicer is multi-functional. It works as a juicer, a food processor, homogenizer, grinder, and a pasta extruder.

This product has a 10 year warranty.

(Information Provided by Amazon.com)

Super Angel All Stainless Steel Twin Gear Juicer - 5500

List Price – $1,200

Rating – 4.5 Stars

Description:

This juicer is a two stage juicer and runs at 86 rpm. It is made from stainless steel parts.

This product comes with a 10 year warranty.

(Information Provided by Amazon.com)

Green Star GS-1000 Juice Extractor

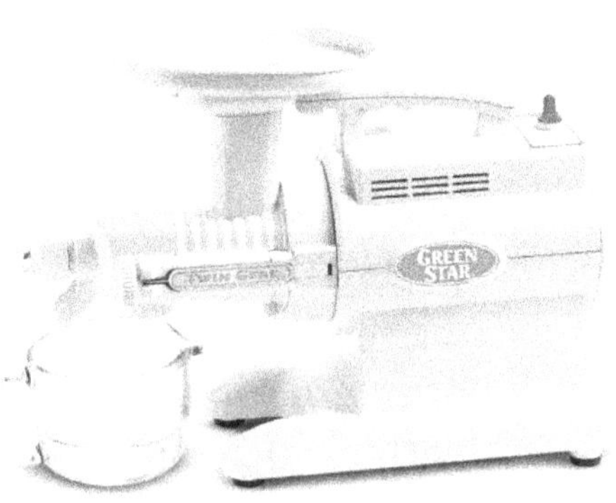

List Price – $529

Rating – 4 Stars

Description:

This juicer has an automatic pulp ejection system which allows for continuous juicing. It can easily juice fruits, herbs, and many vegetables. It can also grind nuts and grains. You can make baby foods, fruit sorbets, and nut butters because it works as a food mill as well as a juicer.

The juicer is easy to clean and easy to assemble. There is a sure-grip handle so that the juicer is easy to carry.

(Information Provided by Amazon.com)

Hurom HU-100 Slow Juicer with Cookbook

List Price – $400

Rating – 4 Stars

Description:

This juicer is known to be able to keep the vitamins and minerals normally found in fruits and vegetables intact. The juicer does not heat up and works at a slow speed, and it runs off of 150 watts of energy.

This juicer comes with a 10 year warranty.

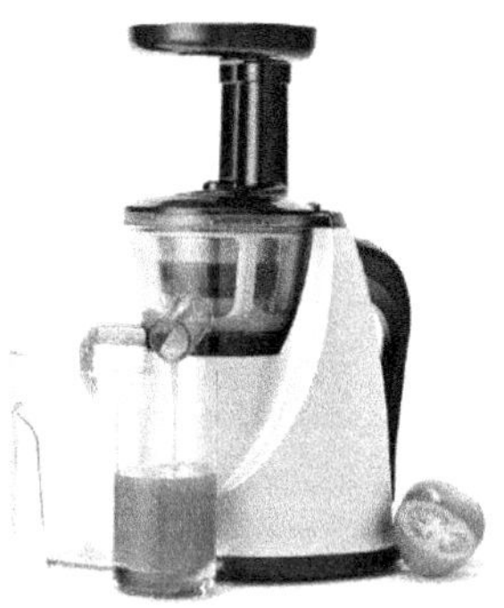

Conclusion

It's All About the Juicy Goodness

Antioxidants and vitamins and beta-carotenes, oh my!

With so many good for you nutrients in our food, it makes you wonder why we don't eat these things as much as we should. When juicing, you're getting the nutrients that your body needs in one shot. Your body is able to absorb the nutrients quicker and you'll begin to feel the effects pretty rapidly—to both your mood and you'll have a little more pep in your step!

It is my hope that now that you are done reading this book, you feel a little more comfortable as you begin your juicing experience. You are equipped with 50 recipes to get you started and some information on the two different types of juicers and the benefits of both types.

Depending on your budget and your needs, you know what kind of juicer best suits your needs.

To keep your taste buds awake and invigorated, make sure that you are using a variety of flavors. It can be a challenge especially if you don't eat a lot of fruits and vegetables as it is. You may surprise yourself though. By trying new flavors and flavor combinations, you may learn that you like things you've never tried before. Who knows, you may even want to eat the new food and not just drink it!

Now, my dear juicing friend, go forth and juice those vegetable and fruits!

www.ingramcontent.com/pod-product-compliance
Lightning Source LLC
LaVergne TN
LVHW010544100826
845148LV00013B/2598

* 9 7 8 0 6 1 5 9 1 8 3 9 6 *